Table of Contents

WHAT IS BELLY FAT?

Abdominal obesity, also known as central obesity and truncal obesity, is a condition when excessive visceral fat around the stomach and abdomen has built up to the extent that it is likely to have a negative impact on health. Abdominal obesity has been strongly linked to cardiovascular disease, Alzheimer's disease, and other metabolic and vascular diseases.

Belly fat is excess abdominal fat surrounding the organs in your stomach. There are three types of fat: triglycerides (the fat that circulates in your blood), subcutaneous fat (the layer directly below the skin's surface) and visceral fat (dangerous belly fat). Visceral fat is located beneath the muscles in your stomach and poses many dangers to your health when there is too much of it.

WHAT CAUSES BELLY FAT

Abdominal fat is caused by several factors including diet, lack of exercise, environmental factors, and genetics.

SURPLUS CALORIES

Poor nutrition habits are the most common cause of abdominal fat.

While it's easy to blame one specific food group or nutrient, like sugar or carbs, for weight gain, the reality is overall calories throughout the week are the real culprit. No matter what you eat, finding the balance of moving your body and nourishing it properly (for the amount of movement you're participating in) can be tricky.

ALCOHOL CONSUMPTION

A systemic review and meta-analysis failed to find data pointing towards a dose-dependent relationship between beer intake and general obesity or abdominal obesity at low or moderate intake levels (under ~500 mL/day). However, high beer intake (above ~4 L/wk) appeared to be associated with a higher degree of abdominal obesity specifically, particularly among men.

METABOLISM

It's easy to blame a sluggish metabolism for weight gain. While it may be true for some, it's not the case for others. There are simple ways to speed up your metabolism if fat loss is your goal.

Metabolism refers to all of the ways in which the body converts fuel for energy. These processes include:

- Breathing
- Circulating blood
- Controlling body temperature
- Contracting muscles
- Digesting food and nutrients
- Eliminating waste through urine and feces
- Functioning of the brain and nerves

You can have a fast, slow, or moderate metabolism—this is largely dependent upon genetics. If you have a slow metabolism it can be frustrating when you're trying to lose weight and it's just not coming off as easily as it may have in the past. Then, there are those with a fast metabolism who can seemingly eat whatever they want and not gain a pound.

Metabolism is also affected by age. Our metabolism slows down as we get older. Many people become less active and as a result, lean body mass (muscle) is lost. Muscle is metabolically active and requires calories to maintain it. If you have less muscle and don't move as much, your metabolic rate will slow down to compensate.

DIET

The currently prevalent belief is that the immediate cause of obesity is net energy imbalance—the organism consumes more usable calories than it expends, wastes, or discards through elimination.

BODY FAT DISTRIBUTION AND GENETICS

Unfortunately, you don't get to choose where your body stores fat. Some people are genetically inclined to store fat in their midsection, while others may store it all over their bodies. In the same sense, you can't decide where you lose fat either.

If you're on a low-calorie diet for too long, the body senses food scarcity and will slow down and store more fat. This is quite the opposite of what individuals limiting their caloric intake often have in mind.

Then, there's something called "familial predisposition," meaning the likelihood of a child becoming obese can be presumed by their family members weight.

HORMONES

Fluctuations and changes within an individual's hormonal health are also associated with abdominal fat accumulation.

Low growth hormone levels as a result of hyperinsulinemia and high cardiovascular risk markers may increase visceral fat accumulation because of reduced sensitivity to lipolysis in this area.

MEDICATION

There are a host of medications that list weight gain as a common side effect. Medications for diabetes, insulin and sulfonylureas, anti-hypertensive medications, beta blockers, corticosteroids, and medications associated with mood disorders, depression, and other psychiatric illnesses have all been associated with weight gain.

Possible Dangers of Visceral Fat

- All-cause mortality
- Cardiovascular disease
- Certain types of cancers
- High blood pressure
- High LDL ("bad") cholesterol
- Low HDL ("good") cholesterol
- Sleep apnea
- Type 2 diabetes

Heart disease

Abdominal obesity is associated with a statistically higher risk of heart disease, hypertension, insulin resistance, and type 2 diabetes (see below). With an increase in the waist to hip ratio and overall waist circumference the risk of death increases as well. Metabolic syndrome is associated with abdominal obesity, blood lipid disorders, inflammation, insulin resistance, full-blown diabetes, and increased risk of developing cardiovascular disease.It is now generally believed that intra-abdominal fat is the depot that conveys the biggest health risk.

Diabetes

There are numerous theories as to the exact cause and mechanism in type 2 diabetes. Central obesity is known to predispose individuals for insulin resistance. Abdominal fat is especially active hormonally, secreting a group of hormones called adipokines that may possibly impair glucose tolerance. But adiponectin, an anti-inflammatory adipokine, which is found in lower concentration in obese and diabetic individuals has shown to be beneficial and protective in type 2 diabetes mellitus (T2DM).

ASTHMA

Developing asthma due to abdominal obesity is also a main concern. As a result of breathing at low lung volume, the muscles are tighter and the airway is narrower. Obesity causes decreased tidal volumes due to reduced in chest expansion that is caused both by the weight on the chest itself and the effect of abdominal obesity on flattening the diaphragms. It is commonly seen that people who are obese breathe quickly and often, while inhaling small volumes of air.People with obesity are also more likely to be hospitalized for asthma.

ALZHEIMER'S DISEASE

Based on studies, it is evident that obesity has a strong association with vascular and metabolic disease which could potentially be linked to Alzheimer's disease. Alzheimer's disease and abdominal obesity has a strong correlation and with metabolic factors added in, the risk of developing Alzheimer's disease was even higher.

What is the best way to get rid of belly fat?

1. Regular exercise is one of the best ways to get rid of belly fat. Aim for half an hour of vigorous aerobic exercise at least 4 times a week: jogging, stationary biking are all great options. Moderate exercises like walking the dog or working in the yard can also help burn belly fat.

2. Following a healthy diet is also an effective way to get rid of belly fat. Diets high in fiber and low in carbohydrates, which include foods like fish, poultry, lean meats, eggs, healthy fats like avocado and olive oil, and lots of colorful vegetables, build up less visceral fat. Be sure your intake of fluids is adequate

3. People who regularly get 6-7 hours of sleep each night tend to have lower measures of visceral fat. Create a healthy sleep schedule for yourself and make sure you stick to it.

FIND WAYS TO REDUCE STRESS

Stress management is important for not only your mental health, but also your physical health. We already know that stress is associated with visceral fat. Finding ways to relieve stress every day can help improve all aspects of your life including disease risk.

AVOID TRANS FAT & HYDROGENATED OILS

Those trans fats on your menu are hiding out in plain sight and sabotaging your lean belly plans every time you eat them. If a food product says it contains partially hydrogenated oils, you're eating trans fat, which can increase your risk of heart disease, high cholesterol, and obesity with every bite.

AVOID EATING AFTER DINNER

Stop treating your kitchen like an all-night diner and you'll stop seeing those unwanted pounds piling onto your frame, too. When you're finished with dinner at night, shut the fridge and don't look back until morning — your belly will thank you. When you do head back to the kitchen in the A.M., make sure the best healthy

FLAVOR YOUR FOOD WITH GARLIC

A little garlic in your meals could mean a lot less weight around your middle. For more flavorful ways to make your food more enjoyable, turn to the metabolism-boosting spicy recipes and watch those pounds melt away.

BRUSH YOUR TEETH

Keeping a toothbrush handy can do more than polish up that smile (and counter the effects of all that belly-slimming garlic); brushing your teeth throughout the day can also help you ditch that belly fat fast. That minty toothpaste flavor not only clashes with virtually every food, but brushing may also trigger a Pavlovian response that tells your brain the kitchen's closed.

Eat More Omega-3s with Fish

If you've got weight to lose and you want it gone fast, try swapping out your usual proteins in favor of fish. Not only is fish lower in calories than an equivalent amount of beef or chicken.

KEEP WHOLE GRAINS IN YOUR DIET

To get rid of belly fat, ditch refined grains like white bread and white rice, and eat more whole grains such as:

- Oatmeal

- Quinoa
- Whole-wheat pasta
- Brown rice
- Barley
- Farro

In fact, opting for more whole grains might just get you there faster.

ADD SOME ACIDIC FOODS

The kind of acid that will help you slim down is the stuff right inside your cabinet., several studies revealed that obese study subjects who made vinegar part of their diet dropped more belly fat than a control group, and other research suggests that acidic foods, like vinegar, can increase the human carbohydrate metabolism by as much as 40%.

SNACK ON VEGGIES

Snacking on veggies is also one of the easiest ways to shed unwanted belly fat, too. Opting for non-starchy veggies, like cauliflower, broccoli, and cucumber, as snacks helped overweight kids shed

17% of their visceral fat while improving their insulin sensitivity over a five-year period.

CONSUME A COMBO OF CALCIUM AND VITAMIN D

Adding some extra calcium and vitamin D to your diet could be the best way to get the flat stomach you've been dreaming about.. To keep your calcium choices healthy, try mixing it up between dairy sources, calcium-rich leafy greens, fatty fish, nuts, and seeds.

RAMP UP YOUR CARDIO EXERCISE

A moderate jog a few times a week can blast through that belly fat.

GET MORE VITAMIN D

While few would suggest you start hitting up the tanning beds for better health, getting some natural sunlight can help you get rid of belly fat in a matter of weeks. To practice safe sun, make sure you're limiting yourself to 15 sunscreen-free minutes per day.

EAT MORE NUTS

Sometimes, to whip your body into shape, you have to get a little nutty. While nuts are high in fat, it's that very fat that makes them such powerful weapons in the war against a ballooning belly.

CUT BACK ON CARBS

Reducing your carb intake can be very beneficial for losing fat, including abdominal fat.

Diets with under 50 grams of carbs per day cause belly fat loss in people who are overweight, those at risk for type 2 diabetes, and women with polycystic ovary syndrome (PCOS).

You don't have to follow a strict low carb diet.

STOP DRINKING FRUIT JUICE

Although fruit juice provides vitamins and minerals, it's just as high in sugar as soda and other sweetened beverages.

To help reduce excess belly fat, replace fruit juice with water, unsweetened iced tea, or sparkling water with a wedge of lemon or lime.

ADD APPLE CIDER VINEGAR TO YOUR DIET

Drinking apple cider vinegar has impressive health benefits, including lowering blood sugar levels.

It contains acetic acid, which has been shown to reduce abdominal fat storage in several animal studies.

Taking 1–2 tablespoons of apple cider vinegar per day is safe for most people and may lead to modest fat loss.

However, be sure to dilute it with water, as undiluted vinegar can erode the enamel on your teeth.

TRY INTERMITTENT FASTING

Intermittent fasting has recently become very popular as a weight loss method.

It's an eating pattern that cycles between periods of eating and periods of fasting.

One popular method involves 24-hour fasts once or twice a week. Another consists of fasting every day for 16 hours and eating all your food within an 8-hour period.

20+ BELLY FAT RECIPES TO HELP YOU GET IN SHAPE

7-Day Meal Plan to Help Lose Belly Fat

Day 1

BREAKFAST

- 1 serving Greek Muffin-Tin Omelets with Feta & Peppers
- 1 medium orange
- 8 oz. green tea

SNACK

- 1 cup low-fat kefir
- 1 cup raspberries, fresh or frozen
- 2 tsp. chia seeds

LUNCH

- 1 serving Whole-Wheat Veggie Wrap

DINNER

- 2 cups Baked Vegetable Soup
- 1 4-inch whole-wheat pita round, toasted and topped with 1/4 cup hummus

Day 2

BREAKFAST

- Greek Muffin-Tin Omelets with Feta & Peppers
- 1 medium orange
- 8 oz. green tea

SNACK

- 1 cup low-fat kefir
- 1 cup raspberries, fresh or frozen
- 2 tsp. chia seeds

LUNCH

- Spinach & Artichoke Salad with Parmesan Vinaigrette

DINNER

- 1 3/4 cups Chickpea Pasta with Lemony-Parsley Pesto

Day 3

BREAKFAST

- 1 serving Greek Muffin-Tin Omelets with Feta & Peppers
- 1 medium orange
- 8 oz. green tea

Snack

- 1 medium banana
- 1 Tbsp. peanut butter

LUNCH

- 1 serving Spinach & Artichoke Salad with Parmesan Vinaigrette

DINNER

- 1 serving Chickpea Curry
- 1 (6-inch) whole-wheat pita bread

Day 4

BREAKFAST

- 1 serving Matcha Green-Tea Latte
- 1 serving Everything Bagel Avocado Toast

- 2 kiwi fruit

LUNCH

- 1 serving Spinach & Artichoke Salad with Parmesan Vinaigrette

DINNER

- 1 serving Roasted Root Veggies & Greens over Spiced Lentils

Day 5

BREAKFAST

- 1 cup kefir
- 3/4 cup unsweetened muesli
- 3/4 cup raspberries
- Top kefir with muesli and berries
- 8 oz. green tea

LUNCH

- 1 serving Spinach & Artichoke Salad with Parmesan Vinaigrette

DINNER

- 1 serving Spaghetti Squash & Chicken with Avocado Pesto

Day 6

BREAKFAST

- 1 serving Matcha Green-Tea Latte
- 1 serving Everything Bagel Avocado Toast

LUNCH

- 1 serving White Bean & Veggie Salad

DINNER

- 1 serving Shrimp Paulista
- 1 cup cooked brown rice topped with 1 tsp. chopped parsley
- 1 cup steamed broccoli florets topped with 2 tsp. olive oil and seasoned with a pinch each of salt and pepper

Day 7

BREAKFAST

- 1 serving Greek Muffin-Tin Omelets with Feta & Peppers
- 1 medium orange

- 8 oz. green tea

LUNCH

- 1 serving White Bean & Avocado Toast

DINNER

- 1 serving Hasselback Caprese Chicken
- 1 cup cooked brown rice
- 1/2 tsp. dried oregano

30-DAY MEAL PLAN TO HELP LOSE BELLY FAT

Day 1

BREAKFAST

- 1 serving Blueberry-Cranberry Smoothie

A.M. Snack

- 1 medium orange

LUNCH

- 1 serving Green Salad with Edamame & Beets

P.M. Snack

- 1 large apple

DINNER

- 1 serving Roasted Salmon with Smoky Chickpeas & Greens

Day 2

BREAKFAST

- 1 serving Apple-Cinnamon Overnight Oats
- 1 clementine

A.M. Snack

- 1 plum

LUNCH

- 1 serving Vegan Superfood Buddha Bowls

P.M. Snack

- 2 hard-boiled eggs topped with a pinch each of salt & pepper

DINNER

- 1 serving Taco Stuffed Avocados

- 2 cups mixed greens tossed with 1 Tbsp. Citrus Vinaigrette

Day 3

BREAKFAST

- 1 serving Apple-Cinnamon Overnight Oats
- 1 clementine

A.M. Snack

- 1 cup low-fat plain kefir

LUNCH

- 1 serving Vegan Superfood Buddha Bowls

P.M. Snack

- 1/2 cup nonfat plain Greek yogurt topped with 1/4 cup blueberries

DINNER

- 1 serving Chickpea & Potato Curry
- 2 cups mixed greens topped with 1 Tbsp. Citrus Vinaigrette

Day 4

BREAKFAST

- 1 serving Blueberry-Cranberry Smoothie

A.M. Snack

- 1 clementine

LUNCH

- 1 serving Vegan Superfood Buddha Bowls

P.M. Snack

- 1 medium pear

DINNER

- 1 serving Buffalo Chicken Stuffed Spaghetti Squash

Day 5

BREAKFAST

- 1 cup low-fat plain Greek yogurt topped with 1/4 cup raspberries and 1 1/2 Tbsp. chopped walnuts

A.M. Snack

- 1 cup sliced cucumber tossed with a pinch each of salt & pepper

LUNCH

- 1 serving Vegan Superfood Buddha Bowls

P.M. Snack

- 1 clementine

DINNER

- 1 serving Slow-Cooker Turkey Chili with Butternut Squash
- 1 serving Guacamole Chopped Salad

Day 6

BREAKFAST

- 1 serving Blueberry-Cranberry Smoothie
- A.M. Snack (164 calories)
- 1/4 cup walnut halves

LUNCH

- 1 serving Slow-Cooker Turkey Chili with Butternut Squash
- 1 medium apple

P.M. Snack

• 1 medium orange

DINNER

- 1 serving Shrimp Cobb Salad with Dijon Dressing

Day 7

BREAKFAST

• 1 cup low-fat plain Greek yogurt topped with 1/4 cup raspberries and 1 1/2 Tbsp. chopped walnuts

A.M. Snack

- 1 medium pear

LUNCH

- 1 serving Slow-Cooker Turkey Chili with Butternut Squash
- 1 medium apple

P.M. Snack

- 1 clementine

DINNER

- 1 serving Polenta Bowls with Roasted Vegetables & Fried Eggs

Week 2

1. Prepare Mini Quiches with Sweet Potato Crust to have for breakfast on Days 9, 10 and 12. Freeze the remaining servings to have in Week 4.
2. Prepare Indian Grain Bowls with Chicken & Vegetables to have for lunch on Days 9 through 12.

Day 8

BREAKFAST

- 1 serving Pineapple Green Smoothie

A.M. Snack

- 1 medium pear

LUNCH

- 1 serving White Bean & Veggie Salad

P.M. Snack

- 1 small apple

DINNER

- 1 serving Salmon & Asparagus with Lemon-Garlic Butter Sauce
- 1 serving Basic Quinoa

Day 9

BREAKFAST

- 1 serving Mini Quiches with Sweet Potato Crust
- 1 clementine

A.M. Snack

- 1 large pear
- 5 walnut halves

LUNCH

- 1 serving Indian Grain Bowls with Chicken & Vegetables

P.M. Snack

- 1 medium orange

DINNER

- 1 serving Flat-Belly Salad

Day 10

BREAKFAST

- 1 serving Mini Quiches with Sweet Potato Crust
- 1 clementine

A.M. Snack

- 1 large pear

LUNCH

- 1 serving Indian Grain Bowls with Chicken & Vegetables
- 1 clementine

P.M. Snack

- 1 large apple

DINNER

- 1 serving Chickpea Curry
- 1/2 (6-inch) whole-wheat pita bread

Day 11

BREAKFAST

- 1 serving Pineapple Green Smoothie

A.M. Snack

- 1 large pear

LUNCH

- 1 serving Indian Grain Bowls with Chicken & Vegetables
- 1 clementine

P.M. Snack

- 1 small apple

DINNER

- 1 serving Vegetarian Niçoise Salad

Day 12

BREAKFAST

- 1 serving Mini Quiches with Sweet Potato Crust
- 1 clementine

A.M. Snack

- 1 large pear

LUNCH

- 1 serving Indian Grain Bowls with Chicken & Vegetables
- 1 clementine

P.M. Snack

- 1 small apple

DINNER

- 1 serving Slow-Cooker Vegetable Stew

Day 13

BREAKFAST

- 1 serving Muesli with Raspberries

A.M. Snack

- 1/2 cup sliced cucumber tossed with a pinch each of salt & pepper

LUNCH

- 1 serving Slow-Cooker Vegetable Stew

P.M. Snack

- 1 small bell pepper, sliced

DINNER

- 1 serving Spaghetti Squash & Chicken with Avocado Pesto

Day 14

BREAKFAST

- 1 serving Muesli with Raspberries

A.M. Snack

- 1 medium orange

LUNCH

- 1 serving Slow-Cooker Vegetable Stew

P.M. Snack

- 1 clementine

DINNER

- 1 serving Charred Shrimp & Pesto Buddha Bowls

Week 3

1. Hard-boil 2 eggs to make Egg Salad Avocado Toast for breakfast on Days 16 and 17.
2. Prepare Brussels Sprouts Salad with Crunchy Chickpeas to have for lunch on Days 16 to 19.

Day 15

BREAKFAST

- 1 serving Apple & Peanut Butter Toast

A.M. Snack

- 1 medium apple

LUNCH

- 1 Veggie & Hummus Sandwich

P.M. Snack

- 1 large pear

DINNER

- 1 serving Walnut-Rosemary Crusted Salmon
- 1 serving Herb-Roasted Root Vegetables

Day 16

BREAKFAST

- 1 serving Egg Salad Avocado Toast

A.M. Snack

- 3/4 cup low-fat plain Greek yogurt topped with 1/4 cup blueberries

LUNCH

- 1 serving Brussels Sprouts Salad with Crunchy Chickpeas

P.M. Snack

- 1 clementine

DINNER

- 1 serving Chicken Fajita Bowls
- 1 serving Guacamole

Day 17

- 1 serving Egg Salad Avocado Toast

A.M. Snack

- 1 large pear

LUNCH

- 1 serving Brussels Sprouts Salad with Crunchy Chickpeas

P.M. Snack

- 1 medium apple

DINNER

- 1 serving Hazelnut-Parsley Roast Tilapia
- 1 serving Roasted Broccoli with Lemon-Garlic Vinaigrette

Day 18

BREAKFAST

- 1 cup low-fat plain Greek yogurt topped with 1/4 cup blueberries and 2 Tbsp. slivered almonds

A.M. Snack

- 1 cup low-fat plain kefir

LUNCH

- 1 serving Brussels Sprouts Salad with Crunchy Chickpeas

P.M. Snack

- 1 medium orange

DINNER

- 1 serving Slow-Cooker Creamy Lentil Soup Freezer Pack
- 2 cups mixed greens tossed with 1 serving Maple Balsamic Vinaigrette with Shallots

Day 19

BREAKFAST

- 1 serving Apple & Peanut Butter Toast

A.M. Snack

- 1/4 cup low-fat plain Greek yogurt mixed with 1/4 cup blueberries

LUNCH

- 1 serving Brussels Sprouts Salad with Crunchy Chickpeas

P.M. Snack

- 1 clementine

DINNER

- 1 serving Eggs in Tomato Sauce with Chickpeas & Spinach
- 1 (6-inch) whole-wheat pita bread

Day 20

BREAKFAST

- 1 cup low-fat plain Greek yogurt topped with 1/4 cup blueberries and 2 Tbsp. slivered almonds

A.M. Snack

- 1 large pear

LUNCH

• 1 serving Green Goddess Salad with Chickpeas

P.M. Snack

- 1 medium orange

DINNER

• 1 serving Sweet Potato Pad Thai

Day 21

BREAKFAST

- 1 serving Apple & Peanut Butter Toast

A.M. Snack

- 1 medium apple

LUNCH

- 1 serving Green Goddess Salad with Chickpeas

P.M. Snack

- 1 medium orange

Dinner

- 1 serving Spring Green Frittata
- 1 serving Guacamole Chopped Salad

Week 4

- Prepare Chipotle-Lime Cauliflower Taco Bowls to have for lunch on Days 23 to 26.

Day 22

BREAKFAST

- 1 serving Avocado Green Smoothie

A.M. Snack

- 1 clementine

LUNCH

- 1 serving Green Salad with Edamame & Beets

P.M. Snack

- 1 medium apple

DINNER

- 1 serving Greek Roasted Fish with Vegetables

Day 23

BREAKFAST

- 1 serving Avocado Green Smoothie

A.M. Snack

- 1 medium orange

LUNCH

- 1 serving Chipotle-Lime Cauliflower Taco
  Bowls

P.M. Snack

- 1 medium apple

DINNER

- 1 serving Sheet-Pan Sesame Chicken &
  Broccoli with Scallion-Ginger Sauce

Day 24

BREAKFAST

- 1 serving Mini Quiches with Sweet Potato
  Crust
- 1 clementine

A.M. Snack

- 1 large pear

LUNCH

- 1 serving Chipotle-Lime Cauliflower Taco
  Bowls

P.M. Snack

- 1/3 cup low-fat plain Greek yogurt

DINNER

- 1 serving Thai Spaghetti Squash with Peanut Sauce

Day 25

BREAKFAST

- 1 serving Mini Quiches with Sweet Potato Crust
- 1 clementine

A.M. Snack

- 1 medium apple

LUNCH

- 1 serving Chipotle-Lime Cauliflower Taco Bowls

P.M. Snack

- 1 clementine

DINNER

- 1 serving Stuffed Sweet Potato with Hummus Dressing

Day 26

BREAKFAST

- 1 serving Muesli with Raspberries
- A.M. Snack (95 calories)
- 1 medium apple

LUNCH

- 1 serving Chipotle-Lime Cauliflower Taco Bowls

P.M. Snack

- 1 medium orange

DINNER

- 1 serving No-Noodle Eggplant Lasagna
- 2 cups mixed greens tossed with 1 serving Olive Orange Vinaigrette

Day 27

BREAKFAST

- 1 serving Creamy Blueberry-Pecan Oatmeal

A.M. Snack

- 1 large pear

LUNCH

- 1 serving No-Noodle Eggplant Lasagna
- P.M. Snack (8 calories)
- 1/2 cup sliced cucumber tossed with a pinch each of salt & pepper

DINNER

- 1 serving Romaine Salad with Grapefruit & Shrimp topped with 1/2 an avocado

Day 28

BREAKFAST

- 1 serving Mini Quiches with Sweet Potato Crust
- 1 clementine

A.M. Snack

- 1 medium apple

LUNCH

- 1 serving No-Noodle Eggplant Lasagna

P.M. Snack

- 1 clementine

DINNER

- 1 serving Vegan White Bean Chili
- 1 serving Guacamole Chopped Salad

Week 5

Day 29

BREAKFAST

- 1 cup low-fat plain Greek yogurt topped with 1/4 cup blueberries and 2 Tbsp. slivered almonds

A.M. Snack

- 1 large pear

LUNCH

- 1 serving Vegan White Bean Chili
- 1 clementine

P.M. Snack

- 1/2 cup sliced cucumber tossed with a pinch each of salt & pepper

DINNER

- 1 serving Roasted Cranberry, Squash & Cauliflower Salad

Day 30

BREAKFAST

- 1 cup low-fat plain Greek yogurt topped with 1/4 cup blueberries and 2 Tbsp. slivered almonds

A.M. Snack

- 1 large pear

LUNCH

- 1 serving Vegan White Bean Chili
- 1 medium apple

P.M. Snack

- 1 medium orange

DINNER

- 1 serving Chicken, Quinoa & Sweet Potato Casserole

SPICY-SWEET GRILLED CHICKEN AND PINEAPPLE SANDWICH

INGREDIENTS

- 4 boneless, skinless chicken breasts (4–6 oz each)
- Teriyaki sauce
- 4 slices Swiss cheese
- 4 pineapple slices (1⁄2" thick)
- 4 whole-wheat buns . Settle on a brand with 3 grams of fiber and fewer than 110 calories per bun.
- 1 red onion, thinly sliced
- Pickled Jalapeños

INSTRUCTION:

1. Combine the chicken and enough teriyaki sauce to cover in a resealable plastic bag and marinate in the refrigerator for at least 30 minutes and up to 12 hours.
2. Heat a grill until hot
3. Remove the chicken from the marinade and place on the grill; discard any remaining marinade.

4. Cook for 4 to 5 minutes on the first side; flip and immediately add the cheese to each breast.

5. Continue cooking until the cheese is melted and the chicken is lightly charred and firm to the touch. Remove and set aside.

6. While the chicken rests, add the pineapple and the buns to the grill. Cook the buns until they're lightly toasted and the pineapple until it's soft and caramelized, about 2 minutes per side.

7. Top each bun with chicken, red onion, jalapeño slices, and pineapple. If you like, drizzle the chicken with a bit more teriyaki sauce.

EASY BREAKFAST HASH WITH SWEET POTATO AND CHICKEN SAUSAGE

INGREDIENTS

- 2 medium sweet potatoes, peeled and cut into 1/4" cubes
- 1/2 Tbsp olive oil
- 2 links uncooked chicken sausage (chicken-apple works nicely)

- 1 medium yellow onion, chopped
- 1 red bell pepper, chopped
- 1/8 tsp cayenne pepper
- Salt and black pepper to taste
- 4 eggs, fried sunny-side up
- Tabasco sauce

INSTRUCTION:

1. Place the potatoes in a medium saucepan and cover with water. Bring to a boil and cook until fork tender, about 10 minutes. Drain.
2. Heat the oil in a large cast-iron or nonstick skillet over medium heat. Cut open the sausage casing and squeeze the meat directly into the pan, discarding the casing. Sauté for 4 to 5 minutes, until the meat is cooked through. Transfer to a plate.
3. In the same pan, add the reserved sweet potatoes, the onion, and red pepper. Cook until the potatoes and vegetables are browned, about 7 minutes. Return the sausage to the pan, season with the cayenne and salt and pepper, and stir to mix.

4. Divide the hash among four plates or bowls. Top each serving with a fried egg and Tabasco.

A VEGGIE-PACKED MINESTRONE WITH PESTO SOUP

INGREDIENTS

- 1 Tbsp olive oil
- medium onion, chopped
- cloves garlic, minced
- 8 oz Yukon gold or red potatoes, cubed
- medium carrots, peeled and chopped
- 1 medium zucchini, chopped
- 8 oz green beans, ends trimmed, halved
- Salt and black pepper to taste
- 1 can (14 oz) diced tomatoes
- 8 cups low-sodium chicken stock (or a mixture of stock and water)
- ½ tsp dried thyme
- ½ (14–16 oz) can white beans (aka cannellini), drained
- Pesto
- Parmesan for grating

INSTRUCTION:

1. Heat the olive oil in a large pot over medium heat.
2. Add the onion and garlic and cook until the onion is translucent, about 3 minutes.
3. Stir in the potatoes, carrots, zucchini, and green beans.
4. Season with a bit of salt and cook, stirring for 3 to 4 minutes to release the vegetables' aromas.
5. Add the tomatoes, stock, and thyme and turn the heat down to low.
6. Season with salt (if still needed) and pepper to taste.
7. Simmer for at least 15 minutes, and up to 45.
8. Before serving, stir in the white beans and heat through.
9. Serve with a dollop of pesto and bit of grated Parmesan.

OVERNIGHT CHIA PUDDING

INGREDIENTS

- 1 cup canned light coconut milk

- 2/3 cup chia seeds
- 1/2 cup plain nonfat Greek yogurt
- 1/4 cup pure maple syrup
- 1/4 tsp salt
- 1/2 cup chopped fresh mango
- 1/4 cup raw coconut chips, toasted
- 1/4 cup chopped macadamia nuts

INSTRUCTION:

1. In a medium bowl, whisk together coconut milk, chia seeds, yogurt, syrup, and salt. Cover and refrigerate 8 hours or overnight.
2. Spoon pudding into bowls. Top with mango, coconut, macadamia nuts, and additional chia seeds.

VIETNAMESE SESAME BEEF

INGREDIENTS

- 450g flank steak, fat removed
- 1 shallot
- 1 Red Capsicum
- 1/4 cup sesame seeds
- For The Marinade
- 2 teaspoons fresh root ginger, grated,

* 2 garlic cloves, minced,
* 1 tablespoon olive oil,
* 1 Tablespoon Brown Sugar
* 2 tablespoons fish sauce,
* 1/4 teaspoon ground black pepper

INSTRUCTIONS:

1. Combine grated ginger, minced garlic, fish sauce, oil, sugar and ground black pepper in a bowl and stir well.
2. Slice beef into half inch pieces.
3. Add the beef to the ginger mixture made earlier. Stir so that the beef is coated evenly.
4. Allow the beef to marinate for a minimum of 30 minutes or preferably 1 to 2 hours.
5. Slice the shallot in thin slices.
6. Slice the red capsicum into julienne strips.
7. Remove the beef slices from the ginger marinade and place into another clean bowl.
8. Add the sesame seeds to the beef and stir to coat the beef evenly.
9. Heat a large, heavy frying pan or wok over a medium-high heat.

10. Once the pan is hot add the onion and fry til aromatic and translucent.
11. Ensuring that the pan is hot add the beef. Do this in small batches as if you overcrowd the pan it will stew not fry.
12. Turn up the heat and stir fry, turning the beef constantly until browned and caramelized on both sides of the meat. Cook only until the meat is just cooked.
13. Remove fro the heat and plate. Serve with a salad

SPANISH GARLIC SHRIMP

INGREDIENTS:

- 1⁄4 cup olive oil
- 6 cloves garlic, thinly sliced
- 1⁄4 tsp red pepper flakes
- 1 lb medium shrimp, peeled and deveined
- 1⁄2 tsp smoked paprika
- Salt to taste
- 1⁄4 cup chopped fresh parsley

INSTRUCTION:

1. Combine the olive oil, garlic, and red pepper in a medium sauté pan set over very low heat.
2. Cook slowly for about 5 minutes, until very soft and caramelized, being careful not to let it burn.
3. Season the shrimp with the smoked paprika and salt and add to the pan.
4. Sauté, turning once, for about 4 minutes total, just until cooked through.
5. Sprinkle in the parsley and serve with bread for dunking into the garlic oil.

WHOLE30 BUTTERNUT SQUASH HASH

INGREDIENTS

- 2 Tbsp ghee
- 1 clove garlic, minced
- 2 cups butternut squash cubes
- 1 cup chopped celery
- 1/2 tsp fennel seeds
- 1/2 tsp minced fresh tarragon
- 1/2 lb Whole30-compliant sausage, or Whole30 Blackberry Sage Breakfast Sausage

- 1/2 tsp salt
- 1/4 tsp freshly ground black pepper

INSTRUCTION:

1. In a large skillet, heat the ghee. Add the garlic and cook until fragrant.
2. Add the butternut squash, celery, fennel seeds, and tarragon, and cook for 5 minutes.
3. Crumble the sausage and add it to the pan with the salt and pepper. Cook, stirring occasionally until sausage is golden and cooked through.

INSTANT POT CHICKEN AND RICE SOUP

INGREDIENTS

- 2 garlic cloves, minced
- 1 yellow onion, diced
- 3 carrots, diced
- 2 celery stalks, diced
- 1 lb. chicken breast
- 5 cups chicken broth
- 1 cup wild rice

- 1/2 tsp dried thyme
- 2 bay leaves
- 1/2 tsp salt
- 1/4 tsp pepper
- 1/4 cup unbleached all-purpose flour
- 1 cup milk
- 5 Tbsp butter

INSTRUCTION:

1. Turn the Sauté feature on the Instant Pot. Once hot, melt 1 tablespoon of butter in the pot. Add the diced onion, minced garlic, carrots, and celery. Cook for three minutes.
2. Add in the chicken breast, chicken broth, wild rice, dried thyme, and the bay leaves. Sprinkle in the salt and pepper, then seal the lid of the Instant Pot.
3. Switch to high pressure (Manual/Pressure Cook) for 20 minutes.
4. When the Instant Pot timer goes off, let it depressurize by itself for 10 minutes. Once finished, release the rest of the pressure from the valve.

5. While the soup is cooking, make a roux on the stove. Melt the other 4 tablespoons of butter in a saucepan.
6. Once melted, sprinkle in the flour and whisk continuously for one minute.
7. When the flour is browned, pour in the milk slowly. Whisk continuously until a thick sauce (a roux) has formed.
8. Remove the bay leaves with tongs from the Instant Pot.
9. Remove the chicken to a cutting board and shred with two forks.
10. Switch it back to the Sauté feature. Pour in the roux into the Instant Pot, then the shredded chicken. Stir until the roux has broken up and a thick soup has formed.

PALEO TURKEY BOLOGNESE WITH GARLIC SPAGHETTI SQUASH

INGREDIENTS

- 1 medium spaghetti squash (2 1/2 to 3 pounds)
- 1 bulb garlic

- 3 Tbsp extra-virgin olive oil
- 1 pound ground turkey
- 1 cup finely chopped carrots (2)
- 1/2 cup finely chopped onion (1 medium)
- 1/2 cup finely chopped celery (1 stalk)
- 4 cloves garlic, minced
- 3 Tbsp tomato paste
- 1/2 cup dry red wine
- 1 (28-ounce) can crushed tomatoes
- 1 tsp dried oregano, crushed
- 1 tsp dried basil, crushed
- 1 tsp fennel seeds, lightly crushed
- 3/4 tsp salt, divided
- 3/4 tsp pepper, divided
- 1/2 cup reduced-sodium chicken broth

INSTRUCTION:

1. Preheat oven to 375°F. Halve the squash lengthwise and scrape out the seeds. Place squash halves, cut sides down, in a large baking dish. Prick skin all over with a fork. Cut 1/2 inch off the top of the head of garlic. Place, cut end up, in the baking dish with squash. Drizzle with 1 tablespoon olive

oil. Bake 35 to 45 minutes or until squash and garlic are tender.

2. While squash is baking, heat 1 tablespoon of the oil in a large pot over medium heat. Add turkey, carrots, onion, celery, and garlic. Cook until turkey is cooked through and vegetables are tender, stirring with a wooden spoon to break up meat.

3. Add tomato paste; cook and stir for 1 minute. Add red wine; cook and stir for 1 minute. Stir in tomatoes, oregano, basil, fennel, and 1/2 teaspoon each salt and pepper. Add broth and bring to boiling. Reduce heat and simmer, uncovered, 30 minutes or until desired consistency.

4. Using a fork, remove and shred flesh from each squash half; transfer to a bowl and cover to keep warm. When garlic is cool enough to handle, squeeze bulb from bottom to pop out the cloves into a small bowl. Add remaining 1 tablespoon oil to garlic. Mash with a fork. Stir mashed garlic into spaghetti squash and season with remaining 1/4 teaspoon salt and pepper.

5. Serve meat sauce over spaghetti squash.

www.ingramcontent.com/pod-product-compliance
Lightning Source LLC
Chambersburg PA
CBHW070047260726
48658CB00002B/771